A Will To Survive
A Womans Journey Through
Chronic Fatigue

A Will to Survive

Lisa Eva Gold

Doctors call what I have, "Chronic Fatigue."
I call it; "A Spiritual Retreat."

"Health is a state of complete harmony of the body, mind and spirit. When one is free from physical disabilities and mental distraction, the gates of the soul open."

— B.K.S. Iyengar

This book is being written with hope.

Hope to inspire those whom do suffer with Chronic Fatigue. This book is based on my personnal experiences and opinions. I am not a Doctor. Everything written in this book is based on a motivation, to survive. An internal drive to move forward in life.

PREFACE

"Clear your mind of Can't"
— *Dr. Samuel Johnson*

THERE IS A STORY about a happy little train. This happy little train rumbled over the tracks on a mission. On a mission to carry her load over the mountain. Her cars had been filled full of toys and good food for girls and boys that lived on the otherside of the mountain. Yet, on her quest, she came to a sudden stop. She simply could not go any further. She tried and tried, but her wheels would not turn. As several trains passed her she would beg for help. In hopes that a stronger engine would hitch on and carry her to her destination. In the end a smaller train that doubted her own abilities, to help, did indeed provide the support the happy little engine needed. The happy little engine did indeed, arrive at her destination.

This is a favorite story of mine. One that I was read too over and over again as a child. Based on the story, *"The Little Train That Could"*, by Watty Piper. It is still my favorite today. The truth of this story is it resembles a "Chronic Fatigue Syndrome". We have broken down. We are unable to carry our load. We have tried and tried. Yet, we just cannot go any further.

But we can.

Hitch on. What have you got to loose? Let us pull each other through this difficult time in our lives. We can do it. As I sit here, my legs ache and my eyes are heavy. Yet, I know we can support each other. If nothing else, may I inspire you to try.

PART ONE

CHAPTER 1

"When you get into a tight place and everything goes against you, till it seems as though you could not hold on a minute longer, never give up then, for that is just the place and time that the tide will turn."
— *Harriet Beecher Stowe*

I AM SCARED. I am so afraid. My body has shut down. My mind, is of no use. I believe this is it. This may be my last phase. I am so uncertain. I feel so powerless. I feel no hope. And I just, do not even have the strength to care .

I awoke with a mission. A mission too write each one of my family members a letter in reference to "my living will". This mission takes me a few days to complete. My strength is weak. Yet, I strive to complete what I feel may be my last mission. I type each letter in reference to my wishes for my body to be cremated, and poured in the ocean. I write each family member my wishes for them to have certain belongings as well as whatever finances left in the bank. I truley feel this is the end for me. I feel sorrow. I feel pain. I feel weak. I place each letter in an adressed envelope. Promising myself that somehow I will get stamps on these letters before my time is up. I place a rubber band around this stack of letters and place this in my night stand beside my bed.

I find myself at home. Alone. I am my own company. It doesn't matter. I don't care. I can hardly keep my eyes open. My 2 dogs lay by my side and my cat on the porch. My daughter is in school and my husband is at work.

I think. I think alot. I wonder why I feel the way I do. I wonder if all my achievements and motivations, have gotten me here. I ponder on the past. And I take a look at my life and all the events that have shaped me. All my experiences, all my lessons, all my mistakes. I truely believe I have burnt myself out.

I reflect on how I got myself here.

I can recall the past year before I became ill. I had worked a night shift position at the local hospital here in Florida. My job was that of a sleep technician. How did I get a job like this? I suppose it had to do with being in the right place at the right time. The opportunity was there. And I took a chance, having no idea what I was getting myself into.

Prior to beginning my new job, an extensive, medical exam and background review, was required. I was to begin my new job on September 12th, 2001. Followed by a required two weeks of on the job training daily. Before, working the required night shift.

I can recall September 10th, 2001 a Monday. My Mother and her husband had flown into New York City. They had plans to stay at Trumph Plaza and then, visit with family, (New York is where I grew up). I had not heard from them on their arrival.

September 11, 2001, we all remember where we were and what we were doing when we heard the tragic news. I recall being so thrilled with my new job opportunity. I had gone to the bank to withdraw some funds for an on-line college course I needed to take for this new job. When the bank teller, looked at me and said, "did you hear what happened?, The twin towers was hit by an airplane." I did not believe what she was saying as I turned to look at the television they had on in the waiting area, I witnessed the second plane hitting the Towers. I sat down and watched the News for a few minutes. I was shocked, just as every one else was.

I had spent my toddler years in Queens, New York. And moved to Long Island with my family when I was eight. In my late teens, I worked in New York city at various different garment companies. I enjoyed my jobs and loved the energy of the city. Now at thirty years old, I sit in my car and am in shock over the events about the 9/11 tragedy.

I wondered if my Mother was ok. I wonder if my family members, and friends whom worked in the city, if they were ok as well. I felt scared, I felt angry, I felt sad. And most of all I felt guilty. I felt guilty because here I am, on cloud 10 thinking about this great new job career, and new schooling I was about to begin. It was a feeling of being this beautiful big ballon, that someone just stuck a pin in, and went........ burst.

I know we all have our stories of this day. And we will never forget it. I did not know what to think or how to feel. I just new that deep down this event really made me think. I cried for the lives lost in such a tragedy. I had not heard from my Mother. Nor was I able to reach any of my friends whom lived in New York. I was no longer excited about my job. I was scared for my well being as well as the American human race.

I did eventually get in touch with my Mother around the 14th or 15th of September since all the phone lines were not working properly. (And I did get in touch with friends). I learned that family members whom did work in or near the Twin Towers did escape safely.

Yet, I felt that regardless of wether we had family members in or near the Twin Towers on this day, it didn't matter. I believe that, we all truley felt the pain of this tragedy. The pain, the lose and the grief. In some way, shape or form, as humans we are all somewhat connected.

We are all people. We have all come from a Mother and a Father. We may have siblings, husbands, wives, children and friends. We all grow up from childhood, with good memories as well as bad. We all do our best as adults to handle responsibilities. Most of us, work jobs in order to pay our bills and supply food to survive on. So, in a sense we are all on a similar path of "life". The difference being; we each have a different road that we must take.

Anyway............ getting back to "my story", of this new job;

I was privlidged with hands on training. And being self motivated, in nine months time, completed the on-line schooling in this field. I had invested and dedicated four and a half years of my life . As I really enjoyed my job and did not mind working night shift. I had a lot of time to pay attention to my patients, as well as time to read. I found myself reading books of interest to me. Through reading I was teaching myself. Learning and focusing more on the spiritual aspects of my life. I read books on Kabbalah, Juidism, and later, included interests in Scientology.

I slept during the days, not paying much attention to the fact that I have a family. And in my off time, I made an effort to attend Shabbat on Saturdays at the local Kabbalah center. Local; being 45 minutes from my home. My husband has different interests and frowned at my motivations. My (now)9 year old daughter, would join me. I think possibly just to be with me, since I was so involved in everything else, ...but my family.

At work, my co-workers were liscenced as Respirtory Therapists as well as Sleep Technicians. I was not. I felt out of place, as well as being treated as "the lesser knowledged one". So, with my motivational thoughts of succeeding, I enrolled in the Respiratory Therapy program at the local college. Already having an Associates degree made it easier for me to get into the program. So, I was not only working night shift 36-48 hours a week, but also attending school full time during the days as well.

Sleep for me? Whats that?

I found the teachers I had were very strict and although I put every intention into study and success, after 3 months of being in the program, I had been encouraged to drop out due to my grades. I beat myself up with my feelings of discouragement, defeat, and lack of success.

At the same time, there was a need for me to also study on my job topics of a Sleep Technician. I needed to focus on preperation for a state exam. An exam that would liscence me as a "Sleep Technician". This required me to take a 200 question exam. The cost of the exam is $300.00. Not including the cost of travel to a town several hours from my home. Nor, did this cost include accomidations for rest, food, etc. Considering my lifestyle at this time, my family would just trot along behind me. We, some how came up with the money to pay for these expenses.

The first exam, for me, being over worked, and overwhelmed, I still had this very stong "Need to pass". However, results proved me, not passing. So, with my ambitions, I had put more time in study and promised myself that I would take the exam again the following year. My family and I came up with the money again. Unfortunatley, again, I did not pass the exam. I was so sure of myself that I would pass this second time around. And when I found out that I did not. I could see red flags go up.

I would think; "Well, Lisa. Maybe this is a sign that this job is, not for you!". I had this overwhelming pressure to succeed.

At 30 years old, I was still trying to impress my family, friends etc, with an "ego status job". I had pressures from my co-workers, and my boss, as well. I had, done all I could do. It just was not meant to be. The stress was overwhelming.

I reflected on the fact that I learned alot and did a good job. The lights were turned on. The lights were burning bright. I realized; I was missing out on the most important part of my life............. My family. They needed me more than this job. I gave resignation, with no agenda to follow through, in terms of having any kind of job.

Yet, when the time came for me to stop working. I panicked. And confided in a friend whom also worked at this hospital, in the Physical Therapy department. And it just so happened to be that she too, was tired of her position at work. She worked during the day as a secretary. And offered for me to take over her position. And in this way, I could still keep my insurance and other benefits with the hospital.

I immediately took her up on the position. Knowing that, I was over qualified for the job and that I would be taking a nine dollar an hour pay cut. At the same time, I deeply felt, and deeply knew, that, being a secretary was not something I wanted to do with my life. I ignored my feelings. And went through with the job transfer anyway.

So, here I was working a day position. Functioning on the same schedule as my family. I liked this. I sleep at night and work during the day. A normal schedule. However...................... I hated my new job.

CHAPTER 2

"For fast acting relief, try slowing down."
— Lily Tomlin

MY NEW SCHEDULE, would begin my day, by getting up and getting my self ready for work. At the same time getting my daughter up and giving her breakfast, and encouraging her to get dressed for school. Which always seemed to be a struggle. I would most of the time forget to eat breakfast myself. As the mornings seemed so rushed. Luckily, my husband has been self sufficant and would usually leave for work, just as my daughter and I were getting out of bed. Some of the time he would take the dogs out before he left for work. Although, many of times, it was just another choir to attend to my busy mornings. I did however, make sure I had some coffee brewing first thing. Don't forget the coffee! And making the beds? Whats that?

So, our "rush" of the morning, leads us out the door. I would drive my daughter to school each morning. As school began for her between 7:45 and 8:00am. My job was less than ten minutes away. As I did not have to clock in until 8:30am.

So, with this short in-between time, I was able to let myself breath. To breath in and just be. Oh, don't think this was an everyday thing. I would like to say it was. But, we were running late many of times. Where I didn't really have time to "breath". And as I would travel to work, I would clench my jaw and dread the thought of my work day.

At the end of the first week at my new job, I requested a meeting with my new boss. Wtih a positive attitude, I thanked her for allowing me this opportunity to work in her department. I also expressed how the major job change and time differences was a stress on my mind as well as my body. I suggested that this postioin was not suited for me. She so proudly smiled and told me what a wonderful job I was doing and how well I seem to "fit in". My ego felt pampered with the praise. And so, again, ignoring my deepest feelings, I told myself, "give it time.............I will adjust."

Yet, my body felt the neglect. When Monday came around again, I awoke with a stiff neck. As I obviously ignored my true feelings of job dissatisfaction, my body took on my negative feelings. This began my, what felt like the,never ending, physical therapy and massage therapy treatments, to ease the tension in my body. Or, shall I just be honest and say to ease the tension of the J-O-B.

In the mean time, I would try and coach myself for work. I would tell myself, "Lisa, just smile". I even bought a motivational CD called "The Joy of Happiness............ at Work", by the Dali Lama. Hoping that this would inspire me to "Like", my job. I would even pray for forgiveness of the dissatisfaction I had for my job. I would tell myself, "Lisa, It is important to remember to be thankful for having a good job. It is important not to take it for granted that it is work under hospital management with excellent benefits, sick pay, vacation time,etc." This speech, however, did not keep me satisfied. I continued to pray for somekind of peace and resolution. A sign of release. I prayed for Something. Anything.

Although this was not my ideal job, it just so happened that I seemed to fit in. I seemed to catch on quick and get the job done. I really liked the people I worked with, and found that, to be, the most important thing about the job itself. Deep down, we know, I hated the job itself. Every day at lunch, I would go sit in my car and cry my eyes out. Not being satisfied with my choices. I felt a bit like if I were in the matrix. My world was just spinning.

So, with my ego in need to succeed, I decided to invest my time and education into "Physical Therapy". I enrolled in a community college an hour from home. I was accepted into the program. I was thrilled. The catch? I had to leave my job. Without any financial assistance, from the hospital or any income for me.

My husband highly suggested that the cost of school was not something we could afford on just his salary alone. I was beside myself! Me, me, me! Like a child. I was so angry. Why couldn't I do what I wanted when I wanted! My ego was deflated, and scared. Scared that I would be stuck with this job position.

Ok. So I am not a quiter I tell myself. I say, " self, in life things happen for a reason". We don't always know why but, we are always in the right place at the right time. Even if we don't see it that way, at the time." I tell myself that possibly with this job I "hate", there is a lesson here to be learned. So, I pretend. I pretend to like my job. I pretend to be as kind as I can to those whom are intolerable, and impatient. I try to play this pretend game. And I keep reminding myself. I say,

"Self, things don't stay the same. Things are always changing. Be patient. The time will come for change." Soon. I hoped.

Four months had gone by with me working in this department. My stiff neck was still a problem, yet tolerable . In the meantime, at home, my husband removed our kitchen, in preperation to replace our cabinets and floors. So, making coffee in the bathroom became routine. And I, personnally did not mind the take out dinners.

In the meantime, I had enrolled in a medical terminology college on-line class. Figuring, that I should just do the best I can with what life offers me. I thought that with the additional knowledge, it would only enhance my work abilities. The course was an on-line computer summer course. If you are familiar with college summer courses, it is a whole semester worth of work cramed into four weeks. No problem, I thought. I could do it. And I did.

In the meantime..............................

CHAPTER 3

"You can't control the wind, but how we sail and navigate is crucial".
— *Lama Surya Das*

I BEGAN HAVING this very uncomfortable feeling around my husband. Like something was just not right. His attitude had changed and he was not pleasant to be around. I focused on the fact that maybe it was not him. But maybe it was me and my anger towards myself in regard to my job success. I still did not have a good feeling around the presence of my husband. Little did I know, what was about to happen............

For about 2 weeks straight every night my husband would be in the bathroom vomiting . I had suggested the hospital. He would argue with me and would firmly state that he did not have a problem. Then one night at about 3 am in the morning, after hearing him vomit for 2 hours straight, I called an ambulance. I felt so scared. I wondered if my husband was having heart faliure. I did not know how else I could help him.

The parimedics took him to the hospital. I had been encouarged to stay home with my daughter at this time. My husband told me that he would call me. So, I tried to go back to sleep. I had work the next day, and my daughter had summer camp. So I called over at the hospital to see what the status was. And there was none. So at around 5 in the morning, my husband called me to tell me he could come home. That he was fine. Ok. So, I picked him up, took him home, and I went to work. It was a Friday.

That night, my husband told me that he did not feel alright and *"asked"* me to take him to the emergency room. His voluntary request to be brought to the emergency room, really had me scared. My stomach was in knots. I could see my husbands face. And his expressions of pain and discomfort. It broke my heart to see him in such pain.

In the emergency room waiting area. My husband was curled up with abdominal pain and had pretty much parked himself in the mens room, hugging the toiet. He is vomiting continuously and crying in pain. I stood by him as we waited close to an hour before he was taken into an examining room. I told the Doctors/nurses on staff, the situation and that he had been treated in this ER this morning and sent home. My husband did not have a Doctor whom he would see regularly, so I requested my family Doctor to see him. After many tests were done, it was found that my husbands pancrease was inflamed. Two weeks later, doctors sent my husband home. With a diagnosis of Pancreatitis only. My husband had been home for two days. When he began throwing up continosouly, again. I took him back to the ER. It was like a de-jevu ER experience that we had only two weeks prior. My husband was re-admitted to the hospital.

My life seemed to be moving so fast. Change indeed. I was exhausted. I did have trouble handling it all. Although I did not express this much at the time. I could tell in my snappy verbal communications with other family members. I could feel my fuse was burning short. Yet, I still needed to try. If not for anybody else, but for my 9 year old daughter, whom all this time seemed to just take it all in.

In the meantime, I had been in contact with my bosses at work. As they were aware of my husband being ill. Thankfully, they were very understanding and alloweed me to work and walk over to see my husband on my lunch breaks and if I was not able to make it to work, they were very understanding as well. This helped, relieve some stress.

My home still was without kitchen. My husbands Uncle hired two of his employees to come into my home everyday and work on assembling a kitchen. I had made time to go to Home Depot to pick out the floor tile, as well as counter tops. (My husband and I had previously picked out cabinets before his illness.)

Each morning I would awake around 5 in the morning. I got my self ready, and my daughter ready for (summer) camp. I made sure that our dogs and cats were taken care of as well. As we leave our home, the two hired men would come in our kitchen, building and assembling. Luckily, my Father-in-law would come into my home and "oversee operations" .

There was so much going on. I felt like a dart board at target practice. Except, the darts never missed the board. They just kept coming at me. I had to remind myself to be thankful. And appreciate the supportive and loving family that were here for me.

After driving my daughter to camp every day, I would go straight to the hospital and sit with my husband for half an hour, before going into work. I found myself not focusing well at work. Although, I put on a happy face, I was really tried of everything. I found myself using my time at work to focus on the on-line college class I had been enrolled in. I did get written up on this. But I really did not care. I was more concerned with my husband recovering. As well as passing this on-line class. Actually, it was good that I had this on-line class to focus on. Because I felt that my whole life was so stirred up, that if I did not find something to focus on, I would completely loose it. I had never had any of my family members terminally ill. And had never experienced having to take care of anyone in my family. So to me this was challenging. As every day after work, I would pick up my daughter from camp and then go back to the hospital where we would eat dinner and sit with my husband until at least 7 or 8 pm.

This was life for now. I was beyond exhausted. I would coach myself on it. I would remind myself that life is a dance. And when it is time to dance.......... just dance. Or shall I say, "Do the Hussel".

CHAPTER 4

"Will someone, open this door and
GET ME OUT OF HERE! ...."
—— *annonymous*

A S MY HUSBAND had been operated on during this
time, Doctors found that he had gallstones. Doctors
removed his gallbladder. And after a total of one
month in the hospital, they sent my husband home. My
husband still did not feel well. After following up with the
Doctor, it had been recommended that my husband follow
up with a outpatient surgery. The Doctor wanted to be
certain that all stones were removed from the gall bladder
duct.

I had taken my husband for this follow up surgery. This
was a successful surgery. As the Doctor did find more stones
in the gall baldder duct. With a sigh of relief, It was now
time for my husband to recover. On this same morning, my
husband, now being at home and able to see our almost
completed kitchen, suggested that "we" go to Home Depot

at the end of this day and pick out cabinet organizers. I suggested that "we" do not do this. Instead, I volunteered to help out and go to Home Depot, come the end of the day.

At Home Depot, I am looking for cabinet organizers. I see up above me, on a shelf, a box with a picture of an organizer on it. I reach up to pull this box out a bit so I can have a better look at the organizer in the picture. Little did I know.....................

The box was not sealed. And therefore the metal contents in this package fell from above and landed on my right foot. Crushing my toes on my right foot. As I screamed and began to cry. I was not sure how much more I could handle. At the same time, my cell phone was ringing. It was my husband calling. I answered it in the state of distress. I briefly explained to my husband what had happened and I needed to find some help and somewhere to sit down. I hung up on my husband. My huband had been recovering from his outpatient surgery that day, as he had been sleeping off the anesthesia.

I finally found a female employee whom found me a chair to sit on. I observed her shaking. And I thought to myself, why is she shaking? I am the one who got hurt. Well, my cell phone rang again, my husband had called me back, in search of me in Home Depot. He came to drive "me", to the hopital. What a nightmare this all has been I think. I can only shake my head and laugh a nervous chukle, at the unfortuante events of my life.

At the hospital, X-Rays had been taken, and although my foot was not broken, the ER Doctor suggested that the injury was bad enough to treat it as if it were broken. I was given crutches and suggested to use them for the next 7 to 10 days. My husband left me in the ER to go pick my daughter up from camp. My husband should not have been driving, considering his recovering conditions. Yet, he picked up my daughter and safely made it back to the ER. I encouraged him to go home with our daughter. That I would be a while in the ER, and that I would call my Mother to bring me home. My Mother had been working and therefore called her husband (my step-Dad), to meet me in the ER. He arrived and waited with me as I was administered,a foot wrap, a special shoe and crutches. Shortly after this, my step Dad drove me back to my home.

Feeling disabled, driving my car was a challenge. As I needed to drive my daughter to and from camp/school. And myself to work. Have you ever had the experience of needing to use crutches? Well, if so than you can agree that it is a workout in itself.

I felt, angry. Like why is all this stuff happening to me? Yet, at the same time, I felt, possibly there is a very big message here that I need to see. The message that it is not a job or school that makes my world go round. But it is my family. It is our health. The biggest thing I needed to see was that, the most important things, I needed to focus on was, "my family". Not my ego, and not my job, and not the additional schooling. I realized that life will constantly throw us curve balls. Yet it is how we deal with them. And whom we consider in the meantime.

I completed the on-line college course. I averged an "A" grade. How I did I do not know. I just did. The grade is not what impressed me most, but the challenge of the "juggle". Feeling invincible............I still hated my job. It was near Christmas time now.

I had set up another meeting with my supervisior. I had expressed to her my gratitude and appreciation for their understanding of my life events. Yet, I still found the job very unpleasant. And I requested a leave of absense. My supervisor, pampered my ego. Again. And I was encouraged to just keep at it. And so, I did.

In the meantime, I had began to not feel well. I frequently had these flu like spells. I found myself calling in sick to work alot. Or, that I needed to leave work early. I new it was flu season. And I just kind of guessed that maybe, my body was trying to fight off the beginning of a flu bug.

It had been the winter holiday season, my favorite time of the year. And the spirit all around was very joyful. For Christmas/Hannukah, my husband had bought me a keyboard. I had played piano for close to 10 years when I was a kid. Being a rebal without a cause, at 15 years of age, I chose not to play piano ever again. Now, at the age of 35 I was just thrilled to recapture the joy of playing an instrument. I could read music. So, it was not long before I invested monies into sheet music that I desired. As I would sit down and play at my convienence.

My husband had also bought each of us a bicycle. I had not riden a bike since I was at least 9 years of age. So, like a child, I was so excited. The next few weekends, my husband and I would set out on Sunday morning, for a 7-10 mile bike ride. Our destiny..........Starbucks.

Piano, and bike riding. Wow, what joy I felt. I felt like a kid again. As I let my inner child, come out to play. I wondered why I took so many years to free myself of restricition. Had I grounded myself, my inner child, without notice? I think of the movie Peter Pan. I relate myself to the character of, being that Peter Pan. Being a grown-up, too strict without cause. And then as we all know one thing leads to another and Peter Pan "gives himself permission" to play again. To be a kid again.

After the 2006 New Year, I had noticed that my black cat, "Spice", was not doing well. She was at least 19 years of age.

And she had been taking medication for hyperthyroidism for a couple of years now. She was my closest companion. We shared so many years together. And we had grown together as well as changed together.

On January 6th, 2006, (a Friday), I had returned home from work. As I noticed Spice, sprawled out on the living room floor. She was barely alive. I immediatly called my husband and told him I was taking her to the vet. He told me he would meet me there.

As it was very obvious, she had already, been on her way to kitty heaven. The loss I felt, was indescribable. I know, those of you who are reading this may think, well, its just a cat. Yet, Spice, was "my cat". And she meant so much to me.

The Vet euthenized her to make her journey from this world to the next, a little more comfotable. I requested that she be cremated. As she now sits in a very pretty small, wood carved box. She is kept at my bedside with pictures of her.

In the next couple of weeks, I found myself still having these flu like episodes. As well, as having feelings of grief that I mourned over my cat, Spice. My family too, had grieved over the loss of Spice. Yet, I do not think that they felt as much of a loss as I did. Then again, it was me that Spice had been connected to for so many more years.

So, life goes on, I would tell myself. I would remind myself of Spice, and considered the long healthy life she had. (Except for the Hyperthyroidism). I would coach myself. I would tell myself that Spice was probably very content in Kitty Heaven, rolling in cat nip.

What a rough year 2005 had been for me and my family. And what a way to begin a New Year (2006). Not to mention that we are Florida residents and also had been affected by the stresses of the Hurricaine season. Alot of grief. Alot of pain. Alot of Change.

PART TWO

CHAPTER 5

"God heals, and the doctor takes the fee."
—— *Benjamin Franklin*

ROUND THE THIRD week of January, I called into work. Unable to get out of bed. I expressed that I indeed had the flu. I did not even drive my daughter to school on this day. I just did not have the strength. The following day, I had called my doctor. I expressed my symptoms and was sure I had the flu. I requested that she call me in a perscription for a flu medication. One that my husband would pick up for me later that day. I scheduled a Doctors visit for four days following. I would be feeling better by then, I thought.

Four days later.........I paid a visit to my Doctor. I was examined and my Doctor commented that, yes my lymph nodes in my neck appeared to be swollen. And more than likely I have the flu and will be able to return to work in a couple of days.

In a couple of days, I still did not feel well. I did however, go into work for a couple of hours. I did not have the strength to do my job. I left work and headed back to see my Doctor. Mind you, I am dressed up and have my make up on. So, as I feel ill, I do not look it. When I meet with my Doctor again, she told me that there was nothing wrong with me. As I disagreed with her, I expressed my thoughts, wondering if I had Mononucleosis. She told me that it didn't matter. Wether or not it is the flu or if it is Mononucleosis, it is still a virus and it will pass. Yet, this "virus", did not pass.

I had requested medical leave from work. My Doctor did not agree that I had any reason to be out sick. My Doctor told me that If I did not go to work that I would loose my job. My Doctor disregarded my ill feelings as being nothing other than a passing virus. My Doctor had not done any kind of blood work. There was nothing to confirm my ailment other than her opinion.

That night, my husband took me to the ER . The Doctors there did a whole blood workup . A diagnosis showed that I indeed had mononucleosis. I did eventually get a medical leave from work. And I did indeed find myself another doctor to follow up with.

My symptoms, seemed to be getting worse. As I would lay in bed at night, I could feel every muscle in body pulsate. An overwhelming achey feeling through out. A feeling of having the flu except ten times worse.

It was a major effort for me to get out of bed and get my daughter to school in the mornings. Most of the time I had my husband or Mother pick my, daughter, up from school. I just could not get myself out of bed. I had to force myself to eat during the days. In the evening, luckily, my husband would cook dinner. As I forced myself to sit at the dinner table, unable to keep my eyes open. I sat hunched over just wanting to go back to bed. All I really had the strength for was to sleep. My eyes heavy when awake, and my body, just a big ache.

The Doctor I did follow up with, suggested I see an Infectious Disease Doctor. When I did, they suggested a recovery rate of six months to one year. They stated that there is no medical cure for this ailment. Yet if I "wanted to try", some different medications, they would write me a perscription. " Perscriptions? Would they cure me of my ailment?", I asked. The Doctors response was, "No". It may help. It may not help". So, why bother I say.

I had made at least 5 visits to the Infectious Disease Doctor. A visit every 3 to four weeks. Each time, I had been offered various different medications to "try". Why were the Doctors so pushy with medications that they are not even sure would help. Besides, being a health nut, I am very big on taking a holistic approach to a cure.

My symptoms seem to remain the same. For what felt like forever. More blood work had been ordered. These tests showed, elevated ranges of a postive "Epstien Bar Virus". I recalled being diagnosed with this, "Epstein Barr Virus",when I was seventeen. At that age thinking I was invincible, I just carried on, regardless of how tired I had felt.

Now, at 35 years old, reality sets in. Finding it more difficult to just, "carry on". I am extremely weak. When I have the strength, I would check my e-mail. As well as go on line and investigate, this mononucleosis virus and epstein barr virus. All results stating, "no cure".

CHAPTER 6

"Take my heart to higher ground.............................."
— *Barbara Stiesand*

I N MARCH, I felt the need to reach out for holisitc healing. I contacted, a healer, Carolyn Cohen. We had met a few years ago at a Kabbalah Center event in Miami. We had kept in touch via e-mail, since our meeting. She had always encouraged me to join in the Healing Circle that was held once a month at the local Unity Church. I just never did.

In contacting her, we scheduled a few healing sessions at her home. She had encouraged me that this illness would pass. She filled my mind, heart, and my soul with hope. As well as positive affirmations that I repeated to myself on a daily basis:

"I can heal myself"
"I am ready to let go.........and let God"
"God is by my side"
"I give God permission to walk by myside at all times"

"I am not alone"
"I no longer need to be afraid of me"
"I am 100% responsible for me"
— *AKA Carolyn Cohen*

"I can heal myself". I want to heal myself without restriction of medications that may cause additional side effects. I want to take a "holistic" approach to heal myself. My mind is strong, yet my body is weak. I have patience. I can allow for a mind, body, spirit, recovery. My mind and body can work together. A mind over matter approach. I give myself this permission. As my mind inspires my body with positive affirmations, my spirit sits in the back seat and gives directions.

In March, Carolyn Cohen and her sister Marilyn Segal were speaking at a seminar, regarding, "Spiritual CPR". Although I was not physically strong, I forced myself to go. In the seminar it was mentioned the importance of prayer, meditation and the importance of keeping a journal. The seminar also inspired us to listen to our minds less. As the mind will frequently, invent unneccesary fears, deferring us from our inner silence, our inner peace.

I had been inspired by the seminar and felt that in some way it would help assisit in my healing process. In the meantime, back at home,my life seemed to be secluded to my bedroom. As my mind kept telling myself, I was getting better. Yet, I seemed to remain, stranded in my bed. I found it difficult to even keep my eyes open to watch tv. My head ached. I had no interests. I hadn't even been interested to opening up a book.

During this time, my daughter was too kind. She seemed to accept the fact that I was not well. Although I felt that it was a difficult time for her. My daughter had come into my bedroom. She said, "here Mommy, I am going to leave this journal here for you, I already have one". Was my daughter trying to tell me something?

Two months had gone by. I had not picked up a book to read, I had no interest. My mind traveled alot as my body stay stationary. The journal my daughter gave me lay next to my bed staring at me. I looked at the yellow journal, with the picture of a black and white striped cat wearing a yellow sweater,sitting in a garden of flowers. Very cute, I thought. Maybe I should begin to journal, I thought. It was something I had always done growing up. Yet, something I did not allow myself time for as an adult. And so I begin to journal again;

March 12th, 2006

Well, its been a long time since I had a journal. Its been a long time since I wrote. Now, I am exploding inside. I have so much to write, so much to say. So many lessons, so many challenges.

Where do I begin- Hmmmm......, ok, I would like to say that I am just going to write like it comes to me whatever mind chatter interrupts, I may just write that down too- "Oh this feels good!" I refuse to be a sealed "bottle", so from here on out I will leave the cap off the bottle. I will, "come out of the closet", as my friend Sara would say.

Ok-life—is a journey as we know. We are to make our corrections in this life time. So trust me, "I HAVE BEEN MAKING THEM".

My daughter, Margo, gave me this journal last week. A few weeks ago, I had given her a journal. So, I thought it was cute that she gave me this . And so I set it beside my bed, and have been staring at it. Thinking what am I going to do with this journal.. But, ok, its cute. Maybe....I should journal again. Nope. Don't feel like it. I went to this seminar last week. And (Carolyn and Marilyn), they

encouraged journal writing. I'm like-it is a good idea, but-----
um...............we'll see.

Anyway, ok, I need an attitude adjustment, "I can heal
myself — I am not alone — God is by my side — I give God
permission to walk by my side at all times — I am 100%
responsible for me — You (me), no longer need to be afraid
of you (me) — You(me) no longer need to hide from you(me)".

I awoke not to long ago. I am laying here to lazy to get up
and brush my teeth and use the bathroom–eventually I will
have too.

So, lets see, hmmmmmmmm............ok, to begin.............I
have been ill with Mono for almost 2 months now. What a
time for healing/cleansing!

Margo, has been so patient and understanding. What a
great kid she is. What a great little person!

So, I've been home in bed mostly since January 18th,
2006. They are expecting me to reutrn to my job April 11th,
2006. If not, then my position will be terminated. Ok- this
does not bother me. What I wonder is what, is in store for me
next? What doors will be opening for me?, what opportunites
lie ahead for me?—'What will I be when I grow up?'. What
will I do for work when I free myself from me? From my
boundaries, and my restrictions — what will become of me
when I see mysef free. I wounder?

I am meeting with Carolyn again on Monday. Her,
influence is powerful. In a good way. I feel she understands
me. I feel like we have an affinity. Its nice to feel understood.

CHAPTER 7

---

*"All your needs are deep within you. Waiting to unfold
and reveal itself. All you have to do, is be still, and take
time to seek for what is within, and you will surely find it."*
—— *Eileen Caddy*

PLACE A meditational CD in the stereo. I sit in my husbands comfortable lazy boy chair. And I think to myself, what a great time to meditate. I am all alone. So, I thought.

I close my eyes. The phone rings. I don't answer it, yet its my Mom so I have to get up and answer it. Ok. So I try this again. I begin by taking the phone off the hook. So, I go back to the chair and close my eyes. My cell phone rings. (ugh). It's my husband, have to answer this one also.

Ok, so, I try this again. I think to myself, I will ignore any types of disruption. This time is for me. So, I sit back and relax. Of course my two small Chihuahas want to get in on this also. So, they too, are sitting with me. Ok. Now to begin.

I sit back, I relax. I take a look around the room. I take a deep breath in, hold it, then release, and take another deep breath in. I close my eyes, and try to clear my mind. Yet, my husband appears in my mind. I have my husband here, (from our brief conversation), and I think these thoughts to go away. Then there is my Mom here, (from our previous friendly conversation). There is the health insurance lady here, the one whom I spoke with on the phone the other day, there is my neighbor, whom always seems to be around when I walk to the mail box. And a dozen other people, I haven't even seen in months. What are they all doing here????!!!. Ok. I say to my self this is got to stop. I am the only one here. This is my head. In my head this is my stage. I am the only one here. So, I say in my head.........."Everybody leave!!!!". Easier said than done. This takes a while. Yet, I do accomplish to do this. Although there is always a peeping Tom like thought that just keeps showing up and repeating nonsense. What is up with that?? Just when I am not thinking a thought, a thought of, nothing matter of fact shows up. Like a distraction. An annoyance. I am sure we all get these.

How strange is this? Why do we feel that our thoughts of the mind, need to occupy every waking second of our lives. And then when we are asleep, well, thats another level of thought thinking. But, could it be that if we don't continue a constant thought process that we think we would some how not be able to function?

It is said, and I have read in various different books, articles, that through mindfull meditation, we find peace. Through meditation, we find our silence. We find ourselves. Focus is the key. To focus on one thing. For instance, when I meditate, I focus on my breathing. The breath that goes into my nose and the breath that leaves my nose. I also at times, may just focus on the rising and falling of my chest when breathing. To focus, on my breath, helps me not to think. As, thinking, most of the time, makes no sense at all and even if it does it is just as if it is a record that just keeps skipping.

As it repeats the same thing over and over again. How funny is this.

Have you ever looked at an animal, dog, cat, bird,etc, and wondered what they were thinking of? I look at my dogs and, wonder. What are they thinking? My one dog knows when it is time to eat, and she will make motion when she needs to go outside to relieve herself. Thats all. If my dogs thought they way humans think, they would not be as docile. Possibly they think of no-thing, most of the time. I wonder if it is possible to think of no-thing? But, to be, at peace in body, mind and soul. At peace with our selves. At peace with our environment.

I recall back in 1990 when I took a Philosophy class in college. It was a great class. Our professor emphasised the importance of meditation. Half of the class time was spent in meditation. I found it so difficult. Yet as the years passed I would always remind myself of this technique.

Carolyin, had asked me if I meditated. "Well, I try", was my reply. My mind is like a little puppy dog. It constantly wants to roam. Where? Anywhere! Anywhere but sit and stay. However, with time and much practice, the phrase, "sit and stay" seems to work for me.

I gather all of the relaxing meditational CD's that I own. And I practice on a daily basis. I find that my dogs also enjoy this time of meditation. As they just seem to mellow in place (usually next to me or on my lap).

Why is it so difficult to focus? Why is it such a task to think of nothing. Like an adult repremanding a child; I tell my mind to sit in the corner and stay. Yet, like an infant, the mind does not like the word, "stay". The mind does not like to be told to be quiet.

In our culture, there is not a big focus on meditation. Why not?

Possibly there would be alot less ego wars. Possibly if we were all to focus on ourselves, there would be less struggles amongst each other. Less, conflict, less chaos.

Possibly.

This reminds me of the song, "Imagine", by John Lennon.

It seems that it has been a never ending battle in our world. A never ending battle for peace and unity. The greatest secret here, is that it starts with us. With me. With you. Where is your peace?

CHAPTER 8

---

*"While praying, listen to the words very carefully. When
your heart is attentive, your entire being enters your
prayer without you having to force it."*
—— *Rebbe Nachman of Breslov*

BEGIN TO pray again. I feel funny doing this. Yet when I was
little, my Mother raised me as a Catholic, so I did indeed
pray before going to bed.

I have this old keep sake chest. My bestfriend in high
school had given it to me years ago. I presently, keep it
hidden in my closet.

On this one particular day, my daughter noticed I had the
chest out of my closet. I opened it, and showed her some of
the special dolls I had collected over the years. There had also
been magazines and newspaper articles of current events in
history that I had kept. As I was going through this keep sake
box, I came across a little box contaning Rosary Beads. The
ones that I had recieved when I had my confirmation at the
age of 12.

Rosary beads. Well, this is a clear enough message for me. It makes me think of my Grandmother, whom always, prayed with her Rosary Beads. I thought, well, why not me? Why shouldn't I pray with Rosary Beads? There seems to be this feeling of having a true connection. Instead of thinking, well, there are millions of people in this world. And how would God know to listen to me. Or, better yet, how would I know he can hear me?

"I have walked to long in the darkness"
—*Barbara Striesand*

Sunday came, I knew I needed to get stronger and I needed Gods help.

I got myself showered, makeup on and hair somewhat fixed. I still felt so weak and just plain strange.

I got in my car and drove to the local Unity Church.

I remind myself that I had been wanting to attend this Church for some time. And now is a great time to begin. This Church resembles a small cottage that I would picture to be out in the woods some where. It is really very cute. Not to big and not too small. Just the right size for me.

And so I am greeted at the door. I enter the sanctuary and find myself a seat. Hoping no one I knew would appear and sit next to me. I was afraid of everyone and everything. I had isolated myself and just needed to keep my space from others. No one sat on either side of me. I actually had the entire row to myself. Ok, this is a good start, I thought.

After service I met, Carolyn and another friend of mine that I had met at the Kabbalah center. I felt at home. A homecoming I had been searching for. I finally found the Church for me. No, not only because my firends were there. But because the service just fit me like a glove.

CHAPTER 9

---

*"Yesturday is ashes; tomorrow is wood. Only
today does the fire burn brightly."*
—— *Old Eskimo proverb*

ENOUGH IS ENOUGH. I tell myself. Tomorrow morning, when I awake, I am going to shower, I am going to put my make up on and I am going to dress as if I have somewhere to go. I tell myself this is my therapy. To stay out of my pajamas, to stay out of my bedroom during the day.

I shall pretend, I tell myself. I have some strength. So today, as well as the next, I shall pretend to feel well. I shall sit in my living room and watch a movie with my daughter. I shall sit on my porch with my 2 small dogs and cat. I shall walk outside and breath in the freash air. And, know that "I" am alive.

Almost six months ago I was diagnosed with what they called, Mononucleousis. Three months later, Doctors call what I have, Epstien Barr virus. And yet, another three months later, Doctors call it "Chronic Fatigue Syndrome".

Shall we place bets? So, what is it.?

And why in the year 2006, there is no cure for this? I have read, somewhere, that this disease has been present among humans since around the 18th century. But what exactly is it? What is the real cause of it? Why do humans get this? Why is there no cure?

> *"It is not good for all our wishes to be filled; through sickness we recognize the value of health; through evil, the value of good; through hunger, the value of food; through exertion, the value or rest."*
> —— *Dorothy Canfield Fisher*

So, what exactly is Chronic Fatigue Syndrome? Is it a sickness? Or, is it a dis-ease of the mind,body and spirit? Wouldn't you agree that this dis-ease is more or less due to our sensitivity in the world? A feeling that we have grown up feeling so different,and at times, so misunderstood. Wouldn't you agree that "Chronic dis-ease", is the way of the body and soul, telling our mind that its time to put on the breaks. Its time to take a look around and appreciate whom we are, and where we are in life.

Regardless of what others may think of us. Possibly it is a time of re-birth. A time of rejuvination. A time to renew our thoughts. A time to renew our attitudes, and motives. Think about this. The mind is very powerful.

> *"God gave me this illness to remind me that I'm not number one; he is."*
> —— *Muhammad Ali*

What has become of me? Who am I ? What has this illness taught me. It seems that I had been on this fast paced road. A road in which, I continuously pushed and shoved to try and get what "I" wanted. Thinking that the path I had been on was the path for me.

Yet, I have learned differently. I have seen that when life's challenges are too difficult, that possibly the road is not for me. Don't get me wrong. Yes, Life has it's challenges. And we have the choices.

Do you remeber the dreams you had as a kid? I do. What did you dream of ? Who did you dream of becoming? What goals as a child did you have for your own future?

What happened to that dream? Did you fulfill it? If so, I congradulate you with trumpets and honors. If, not............... why not? What got in your way of reaching your goals?

When I was a kid, I would joke around and say that I would be going out to look for myself. I can tell you that through my illness, through this journey, through this time of re-awakening, I have found myself. I have been here all along.

I have given myself permission to be. Permission to take off the "knights" silver armour. I give myself this permission to see the light. And to set myself free of me. To not fight in a war against myself. To allow myself the freedom that has always been there. Yet, I had been too blind to see. To confused, by trying to keep up with everyone else.

Yet, being on so many different roads during my life, has taught me so many lessons.

For every posivite lesson I have learned is like a feather added into my invisible back pak. And for every negative lesson learned, has been a rock added into my invisible back pak. Possibly it is through this illness. That I have emptied out this invisible back pak. So, I may no longer carry such a heavy sack. As a result, my body aches may be relieved.

In carrying a lighter load, my focus becomes clear. I can see that my family is whom I need to impress, not my boss. I see that what I need to work on is my behavior here at home. My attitude, my actions, my deeds. All begin here at home. As a Mother, as a Wife, I am important to me. I am important to my family. It is here, that I learn the most. It is at home that "I", affect and am affected by.

I have read, and I have heard it said; that our destiny cannot be changed. Yet, the roads in which we take in getting there has it's challenges. It is our attitude and our motives that shape our way. That shape who we are and prepare us for what lies ahead.

It seems so strange. I feel so different. I find me to be a stranger in a strange land. As I come in contact with others in public places, be it the grocery store, etc.; I seem to be able to see through other people. I can see the irritation in their faces. I can see stress oozing out of thier pores. I can feel their unhappiness. I find that there are so many very unhappy people in this world. Am I the only one that feels at peace with my self?

At the store, I approach a cashier at a store to check out. I feel as though the cashier looks at me as if I am some alien form another planet. Is it me I wonder? I do not believe so. Yet, I am not perfect. Did I say something out of line? Was I not polite enough? Or was I too polite?

Well, I could just drive myself nuts wondering why I do not fit in with the rest of the world. Maybe, I should just stop trying to fit in and allow myself to just be. Why do we try so hard to fit in? Why do we try so hard to please others and please ourselves last? Would you agree that we should focus more on our own needs rather than focus on others needs?

This makes me more thankful for the few friends and the loving family that I do have. Yet it also makes me feel so very small. That there are just so few of us. So few who understand what I see, and who feel what I feel. Call it psychic abilities. Or call me insane. Either way, I still remain, "sitting on the fence."

So with much love, I wish you all the best in your recovery..............

A NEW BEGINNING

I truely believe it is possible to live several lives in the existing body to which we are contand in. It is all a matter of what mind set we keep and what we change about ourselves. It is not so much that the world changes around us, but more so, it is our view that changes.

Since I have written this book, I have realized how much I tried to build my world around my husband. How his unhealthy, controlling, habits had such an influence on my existance. It is not so important to know what his controlling, addictive habits were. But it is more important to realize that a healthy relationship, is one that allows you to grow as an individual and not as a prisioner. I had been a prisioner, in more ways than mentioned in this book.

I am now divorced, and living with my daughter. I am healthy and I am happy. Making healthy decisions, I presently own my own business teaching piano. I am so very thankful for all that I have in my life as well as my family and friends. Without such support, I don't know if I would be where I am today. I feel so very blessed. And most of all, I am thankful for my daughter. For she teaches me so much.

Yet, more so, than this. I have survived. I have over come what they call Chronic Fatigue. I have overcome this through a will to survive. The will to continue to move forward. To realize that each day lived is not the same. That each day brings with it new lessons, new experences. What a gift it is to be alive and well.

There is no cure for Chronic Fatigue. Possibly what Chronic Fatigue really is, is a wake up call. Our own bodies telling us, enough is enough. Possibly Chronic Fatigue is a retreat. A time for us to shut down, and take a better look at ourselves, our lives. A step back from life in order to rearrange and prioritize our life. This is what I have done. And with a will to survive, my mind continues to grow stronger and wiser. To realize that life does not need to be so challenging and difficult. That we are all 100% in controll of our selves and the decisions we make. I have decided to be healthy. And so it is...................

The story in which I have shared with you is one of many of my stories.

RECOMMENDED READINGS:

–*"Whose Illness is is Anyway?/ A Mystical Journey to Wellness"*
by Marilyn Segal and Carolyn Cohen

–*"Heal Your Body"*
by Louise L. Hay

–*"Complete Aromatherapy Handbook/Essential Oils for Radiant Health"*
by Susanne Fischer–Rizzi

–*"Break Through Pain/Intergrated CD Learning"*
by Shinzen Young

–*"Healing Trauma/ A Pioneering Program for Restoring the Wisdom of Your Body/Intergrated CD Learning"*
by Peter A. Levine, PH.D

–*"The Artisit's Way/A Spiritual Path To Higher Creativity"*
by Julia Cameron

–*"The Power of Now/A guide to Spiritual Enlightenment"*
by Eckhart Tolle

-*"Talking to Heaven"*
by James Van Praagh

-*"Reaching to Heaven"*
by James Van Praagh

-*"Heaven and Earth"*
by James Van Praagh

-*"Healing Grief/Reclaiming Life After Any Loss"*
by James Van Praagh

-*"The Seat of the Soul"*
by Gary Zukav

-*"Letting Go of the Person You Used to Be"*
by Lama Surya Das

-*"No Death, No Fear/Comforting Wisdom for Life"*
by Thich Nhat Hanh

-*"An Open Heart/Practicing Compassion in Everyday Life"*
by The Dalai Lama

-*"Same Soul Many Bodies"*
by Brian L. Weiss, M.D.

Recommended CDs':

SWEET SERENITY
by Eloiwa DeFreitas
GUIDED MEDITATION
by Kelly Howell

DEEP MEDITATION
by Kelly Howell

HOW THE HEAVENS HEAL
with Karen Berg

HIGHER GROUND
by Barbara Streisand

TRUST YOUR VIBES/SECRET TO SIX–SENSORY LIVING
by Sonia Choquette

YOUR PSYCHIC PATHWAY/LISTENING TO THE GUIDING WISDOM OF YOUR SOUL
    by Sonia Choquette

INFINITE SELF/33 STEPS TO RECLAIMING YOUR INNER POWER
by Stuart Wilde

DISSOLVING BARRIERS
by Louise L. Hay

OVERCOMING FEARS/CREATING SAFETY FOR YOU AND YOUR WORLD
    by Louise L. Hay

FORGIVNESS/LOVING THE INNER CHILD
by Louise L. Hay
CAROLINE MYSS'/CHAKRA MEDITATION MUSIC
by Steven McNamara

The Mindbody Prescription/Healing the Body, Healing the Pain"
    by John E. Sarno, M.D.

Recommended Web–Sites:

Healing Facilitator;
Sky@AngelicRetreats.com
www.AngelicRetreats.com
Healing from the Inside Out
TwinWisdom.com
Soul Healing & Medical Intuit;
clcohen2@yahoo.com
Life Purpose & Coaching;
marilynsegal@bellsouth.net

Recommended Viewing:
"BE STILL/ And know that I am God ....Psalms 46:10"
DVD
"THE SECRET"
DVD

www.ingramcontent.com/pod-product-compliance
Lightning Source LLC
Chambersburg PA
CBHW070336290526
45791CB00003B/1352